CBD OIL GUIDE

BOB MARLEY

THE HEALTH BENEFITS OF CBD OIL AND HOW TO USE IT FOR NATURAL HEALING

TABLE OF CONTENTS

TABLE OF CONTENTS..

INTRODUCTION ....

CHAPTER 1 ....

    HOW CBD BENEFITS THE BODY ....

CHAPTER 2 ....

    HOW DOES CBD WORK IN THE BODY..

    CHAPTER 3 ....

THE ENDOCANNABINOID SYSTEM..

CHAPTER 4 ....

    WHAT IS CBD HEMP OIL ....

CHAPTER 5 ....

    CBD OIL FOR DIABETES ....

CHAPTER 6 ....

    CBD HEMP OIL CURES EPILEPSY ....

CHAPTER 7 ....

    CBD HEMP OIL HARDENS BONE...

CHAPTER 8 ....

    CBD HEMP OIL CURES BACK PAIN ....

CHAPTER 9 ....

    CBD HEMP OIL CURES ARTHRITIS..

CHAPTER 10 ....

    CBD HEMP OIL CURES FIBROMYALGIA ....

CHAPTER 11 ....

    CBD HEMP OIL CURES SCLEROSIS..

CHAPTER 12 ....

    IS CBD HEMP OIL LEGAL?..

CHAPTER 13 ....

    WHAT ARE THE VARIOUS TYPES OF HEMP OIL ....

CHAPTER 14 ....

    THINGS TO CONSIDER WHEN BUYING HEMP SEED OIL.........................

CHAPTER 15 ....

    HOW DO YOU MAKE CBD HEMP OIL ....

CHAPTER 16 ....

    HOW YOU CAN USE HEMP OIL FOR HEALTH AND BEAUTY?.................

SUMMARY...

INTRODUCTION

CBD is one of over 60 compounds found in cannabis that belongs to a class of ingredients called cannabinoids. Until recently, THC (tetrahydrocannabinol) was getting most of the attention because it's the ingredient in cannabis that produces mind-altering effects in users, but CBD is also present in high concentrations, and the medical world is realizing that its list of medical benefits continues to grow.

Cannabidiol, or CBD as it is commonly known, is a very interesting chemical; it is responsible for many people changing their views on

7

marijuana use for medicinal purposes. While everyone has heard of THC, not many are aware of CBD; the two chemicals are both contained in marijuana but they serve very different purposes. While the THC in marijuana is going to get you high, CBD is something that poses huge benefits from a medicinal point of view, and it does not have the same side effects on the body as THC.

Here are some facts to know about CBD;

1. KEY INGREDIENT IN CANNABIS

When we look at the main ingredients in cannabis, we immediately note the relevance of THC and CBD. These chemicals are present in the highest concentrations in cannabis crop, no matter how it is grown. Even recreational marijuana breeders have noticed that there are high levels of CBD in their crop. Some have even managed to grow cannabis with a lot of CBD but very little THC, and these strains are becoming more and more popular each year because people want the benefits of CBD without the negative side-effects of THC.

2. **CBD IS NOT PSYCHOACTIVE**

Contrary to popular belief, products such as CBD oil or CBD capsules are not going to get you high. The CBD in these products, or the CBD you find in cannabis, is not going to make you feel the same as the THC does. It is THC that is a psychoactive substance while CBD is not. It does not act in the same manner when it comes into contact with your brain's pathways, it does not interfere with your psychomotor or psychological functions either. For those who want a simpler explanation, CBD is 100 percent safe and is not going to get you high!

3. **MEDICAL BENEFITS**

There are many different health benefits to taking CBD; for example, it can help people who are experiencing excessive nausea and vomiting because they are going through chemotherapy or some other type of treatment. It is also great at suppressing the seizures some people get on a regular basis. Another benefit to CBD is how it

9

helps combat inflammation and neurodegenerative disorders. It is also great for depression and anxiety sufferers. So if you are suffering from one of these conditions, you may want to talk to your physician about the possibility of getting CBD oil or CBD capsule supplements for a few months.

4. **CBD LIMITS THC EFFECTS**

It is interesting to note that the strains of cannabis that contain a lot of THC are the ones that cause people to feel sleepy, disoriented and "high." Many users who use the cannabis strains that contain a high amount of CBD comment that they do not suffer the same symptoms, in fact, some claim to feel more alert. The alertness comes due to the fact that the CBD is counteracting the impact of the THC on the body, rendering those strains of cannabis relatively harmless too.

CHAPTER 1

HOW CBD BENEFITS THE BODY

1. RELIEVES PAIN AND INFLAMMATION

Among common CBD benefits, natural pain relief tops the list for many. Evidence suggests that cannabinoids may prove useful in pain modulation by inhibiting neuronal transmission in pain pathways. A 2012 study published in the Journal of Experimental Medicine found that CBD significantly suppressed chronic inflammatory and neuropathic pain in rodents without causing analgesic tolerance. Researchers suggest that CBD and other nonpsychoactive components of marijuana may represent a novel class of therapeutic agents for the treatment of chronic pain.

According to a 2007 meta-analysis conducted in Canada, the combination of CBD and THC buccal spray was found to be effective in treating neuropathic pain in multiple sclerosis, which can be debilitating for 50 to 70 percent of MS patients.

2. HAS ANTIPSYCHOTIC EFFECTS

Research shows that CBD benefits include producing antipsychotic effects; it appears to have a pharmacological profile similar to that of a typical antipsychotic drugs as seen using behavioral and neurochemical techni□ues in animal studies. Additionally, studies show that CBD prevents human experimental psychosis and is effective in open case reports and clinical trials in patients with schizophrenia, with a remarkable safety profile.

3. REDUCES ANXIETY

Studies using animal models of anxiety and involving healthy volunteers clearly suggest an anxiolytic-like effect of CBD.

Cannabidiol has shown to reduce anxiety in patients with social anxiety disorder and researchers suggest that it may also be effective for panic disorder, obsessive compulsive disorder, social anxiety disorder and post-traumatic stress disorder.

A 2011 study aimed to compare the effects of a simulation public speaking test on healthy control patients and treated native patients with social anxiety disorder. A total of 24 never-treated patients with social anxiety disorder were given either CBD or placebo 1.5 hours before the test. Researchers found that pretreatment with CBD significantly reduced anxiety, cognitive impairment and discomfort in their speech performance, and significantly decreased alertness in anticipation of their speech; the placebo group presented higher anxiety, cognitive impairment and discomfort.

4. HELPS TO FIGHT CANCER

Several scientific reports demonstrate that CBD benefits include possessing antiproliferative, pro-apoptotic effects that inhibit cancer cell migration, adhesion and invasion. A 2006 study published in the Journal of Pharmacology and Experimental Therapeutics found for the first time that CBD potently and selectively inhibited the growth of different breast tumor cell lines and exhibited significantly less potency in non-cancer cells.

In 2011, researchers added light on the cellular mechanism through which CBD induces breast cancer cells; they showed that CBD induced a concentration-dependent cell death of both oestrogen receptor-positive and oestrogen receptor-negative breast cancer cells. They also found that the effective concentrations of CBD in tumor cells have little effect on non-tumorigenic, mammary cells.

CBD behaves as a non-toxic compound, and studies show that doses of 700 milligrams per day for 6 weeks did not show any overt toxicity in humans, suggesting that it can be used for prolonged treatment. Not only does the research show that CBD benefits include being effective in fighting breast cancer cells, data also

15

suggests that it can be used to inhibit the invasion of lung and colon cancer, plus it possesses anti-tumor properties in gliomas, and has been used to treat leukemia.

5. RELIEVES NAUSEA

Cannabis has been used for centuries for the suppression of nausea and vomiting. Research has revealed that among more than 80 cannabinoid compounds found in marijuana, both the intoxicant THC and the non-intoxicant CBD helps to get rid of nausea and vomiting in animal studies. A 2012 study published in the British Journal of Pharmacology found that CBD benefits included possessing anti-nausea and antiemetic effects, which was discovered when it was administered to rats. Researchers found that CBD acts in a diphasic manner, meaning that in low doses, it suppresses toxin-induced vomiting, but in high doses it increases nausea or has no effect.

6. MAY TREAT SEIZURES AND OTHER NEUROLOGICAL DISORDERS

A 2014 survey conducted by researchers at Stanford University was presented to parents belonging to a Facebook group dedicated to sharing information about the use of cannabidiol-enriched cannabis to treat their child's seizures. Nineteen responses met the inclusion criteria for the study: a diagnosis of epilepsy and current use of CBD-enriched cannabis.

The average number of anti-epileptic drugs tried before using CBD cannabis was 12. Sixteen (84 percent) of the 19 parents reported a reduction in their child's seizure frequency while taking CBD cannabis; Of these, two (11 percent) reported complete seizure freedom, eight (42 percent) reported a greater than 80 percent reduction in seizure frequency, and six (32 percent) reported a 25–60 percent seizure reduction. Other beneficial effects included increased alertness, better mood and improved sleep; while side effects included drowsiness and fatigue.

Later in 2014, researchers reported the preliminary results of a study involving children with treatment-resistant epilepsies in an expanded access "compassionate use program." Patients received a purified 98 percent oil-based CBD extract called Epidiolex, which is made by GW Pharmaceuticals. After 3 months of treatment, 39 percent of the 23 patients had more than a 50 percent reduction in seizures, with a 32 percent median reduction. These preliminary results support the animal studies and survey reports that CBD may be a promising treatment for treatment-resistant epilepsy and it is generally well-tolerated in doses up to 25 milligrams per kilogram of body weight.

7. LOWERS INCIDENCE OF DIABETES

A 2006 study found that CBD treatment significantly reduced the incidence of diabetes in non-obese diabetic mice from an incidence of 86 percent in non-treated mice to an incidence of 30 percent in CBD-treated mice. CBD benefits also showed a significant reduction of plasma levels of pro-inflammatory cytokines. A histological examination of the pancreatic islets of the CBD-treated mice revealed significantly reduced insulitis.

In 2013, the American Journal of Medicine published a study that highlighted the impact of marijuana use on glucose, insulin and insulin resistance among U.S. adults. The study included 4,657 adult men and women from the National Health and Nutritional Examination Survey from 2005 to 2010; of the participants, 579 were current marijuana users and 1,975 were past users. The researchers found that current marijuana use was associated with 16 percent lower fasting insulin levels. They also found significant associations between marijuana use and smaller waist circumferences, a factor connected to the onset of diabetes symptoms.

8. PROMOTES CARDIOVASCULAR HEALTH

A 2013 study published in the British Journal of Clinical Pharmacology reports that CBD protects against the vascular damage caused by a high glucose environment, inflammation or the induction of type 2 diabetes in animal models; plus, CBD proved to reduce the vascular hyperpermeability (which causes leaky gut) associated with such environments.

CHAPTER 2

HOW DOES CBD WORK IN THE BODY

Like all cannabinoids, CBD interacts with your body through its native endocannabinoid system, or ECS. Present in all mammalian species, including humans, the endocannabinoid system is a complex signaling network responsible for establishing and maintaining health by regulating many of the body's natural functions, including mood, memory, appetite, pain, immune response and temperature.

The endocannabinoid system is made up of cannabinoid receptors and substances called endocannabinoids, which according to Medscape are synthesized by the body on demand. The cannabinoid receptors found throughout the body, work like a lock and key to bind with endocannabinoids.

When the endocannabinoids bind or interact with these receptors, they alter the release of neurotransmitters to relay messages between nerve cells. The endocannabinoid system is constantly using endocannabinoids and cannabinoid receptors to make the necessary adjustments to keep our many functions in a general state of balance.

Plant-derived cannabinoids like CBD, found in hemp and marijuana, mimic many of the biological actions of the endocannabinoids that are synthesized by the body. Like endocannabinoids, CBD interacts with the cannabinoid receptors as the endocannabinoid system works to keep the body and its functions in homeostasis.

Thousands of studies have been done investigating CBD and the natural balancing effects from its interaction with the endocannabinoid system.

CHAPTER 3

THE ENDOCANNABINOID SYSTEM

THE CB1 AND CB2 RECEPTORS

Cannabinoid receptors are involved in a series of processes inside the human body, including the regulation of mood, pain sensation, appetite and memory. These receptors can be activated by endocannabinoids (produced by the human body) as well as by plant cannabinoids (like those found in hemp or cannabis), and they are grouped in two main categories: CB1 and CB2.

CB1 receptors are found mostly in the central nervous system and in smaller numbers in the liver, kidneys and lungs; while CB2 receptors are part of the immune system and found in the hematopoietic blood cells. CB1 plays a role in the production and release of neurotransmitters, cannabis products that exert psychoactive effects stimulate these receptors.

At the same time, CB1 receptors are involved in the lipogenesis process that takes place inside the liver, and seem to play a role in the maintenance of homeostasis (body's internal e□uilibrium). Various studies suggest that CB1 also influences pleasure, concentration and appetite, memory and pain tolerance.

CB2 receptors on the other hand affect the immune system, being involved in a variety of functions like immune suppression or apoptosis (programmed cell death). Studies suggest that CB2 modulate the pain sensation and could play a role in various diseases, from liver and kidney problems to neurodegenerative diseases.

CBD does not stimulate these two receptors; instead, it activates other receptors, like the vanilloid, adenosine and serotonin receptors. By activating the TRPV-1 receptor for example, cannabidiol plays a role in the mediation of body temperature, pain perception and inflammation. Then, CBD inhibits the FAAH enzyme, a compound that activates the CB1 receptor; by doing so, CBD minimizes the activation of CB1 by THC, reducing its psychoactive effects.

The activation of adenosine receptors by CBD gives the anti-anxiety and anti-inflammatory effects of cannabidiol. Adenosine receptors are also involved in the release of dopamine and glutamate, two neurotransmitters that play major roles inside the body. Dopamine is involved in cognition, motor control, motivation and reward mechanisms, while glutamate is one of the major mediators of excitatory signals, being involved in memory, learning and cognition.

High concentrations of CBD have been shown to activate the 5-HT1A serotonin receptor, exerting anti-depressant effects. The same receptor is involved in a series of processes from pain perception, appetite, nausea and anxiety to sleep and addiction mechanisms.

Finally, CBD blocks CPR55 signaling, decreasing bone re-absorption and cancer cell proliferation. GPR55 is widely present inside the brain, being linked with the modulation of bone density and blood pressure, as well as with cancer cell proliferation.

As previously said, CBD blocks the psychoactive action of THC, this being one of the reasons it is generally considered advantageous to combine CBD and THC for treatment purposes. However, the positive effects of cannabidiol are not dependent on the presence of THC, so you can still take advantage of the health benefits of CBD by purchasing products that contain only non-psychoactive CBD.

CHAPTER 4

WHAT IS CBD HEMP OIL

Derived from the stalk and seed of cannabis (hemp) plants, cannabidiol (CBD) oil or CBD hemp oil is a natural botanical concentrate that is high in the compound CBD. Of the more than 85 cannabinoids so far identified in the cannabis plant, CBD is the second most common after tetrahydrocannabinol (THC). Unlike THC, CBD is non-psychotropic and therefore doesn't cause a euphoric high.

Pure CBD hemp oil is extracted from the cannabis varieties that are naturally abundant in CBD, and low in THC. A specialized extraction process is used to yield highly concentrated CBD oil or pure cannabidiol that also contains other nutritious material such as omega-3 fatty acids, terpenes, vitamins, chlorophyll, amino acids, and other phytocannabinoids like cannabichromene (CBD), cannabigerol (CBG), cannabinol (CBN) and cannabidivarian (CBCV).

Pure hemp cannabidiol oil can be consumed directly as a nutritional supplement. Over the years, great advances in CBD hemp oil product development have led to what are now dozens of different types of CBD hemp oil products, including capsules, drops, and even chewing gum. Concentrated pure CBD hemp oil can also be infused into skin and body care products and used topically.

Our understanding of CBD cannabis oil has expanded and we're more aware today than ever of the cannabinoid's potential. Studies on CBD's natural health benefits are extensive and groundbreaking research is being done regularly. We suggest you review the wide body of scientific research on CBD to get a better understanding of the cannabinoid's health value.

CHAPTER 5

CBD OIL FOR DIABETES

Diabetes is a disease wherein the body has trouble regulating the level of sugar (glucose) in the bloodstream. In healthy individuals, the pancreas produces a hormone called insulin, which works to transport glucose molecules across cell membranes and into cells for energy production.

In diabetics, depending on whether they suffer from the Type 1 or Type 2 form of the disease, the body is either unable to produce insulin, or it's unable to use it in a way that's sufficient enough to maintain glucose at a healthy level in the bloodstream.

In turn, irregular or unstable glucose levels can cause a huge array of serious, life threatening conditions, which we'll talk about in detail shortly.

In regard to CBD oil for diabetes, then, there are two main things we need to consider in order to determine the degree of viability that the drug has on the increasingly-prevalent disease:

In what ways (if any) does CBD work to improve either the function and/or production of insulin, and

How does CBD work to alleviate the spectrum of side effects caused by irregular blood sugar levels.

In this chapter, we'll talk about recent research publications which directly address both of these questions, in the hopes of shedding some light on why CBD oil for diabetes is gaining such popularity among both patients and physicians alike.

DIABETES: WHAT IS IT, WHAT CAUSES IT, AND WHO IS AT RISK

To elaborate on the rudimentary processes explained in the introduction, diabetes is a disease wherein the body is unable to properly transfer the glucose from food into energy sources for cells.

And of course, without energy sources, the body's cells (which are responsible for every functional mechanism of life) will be unable to carry out the re□uisite pathways needed to survive.

In the case of Type 1 diabetics (who only make up about 5% of the diabetic population), the body is no longer able to produce insulin, which is the keystone hormone needed to transfer glucose molecules from the bloodstream into cells. This is generally due to an autoimmune attack on the pancreas – the organ responsible for the production of insulin. Type 1 diabetes usually arises in children or young adults who contract a pancreas-attacking virus, and other than perhaps a genetic predisposition, there are not many specific risk factors.

Type 2 diabetes is a rather more complex form of the disease wherein the body still produces insulin, but it either doesn't produce enough of it, or the cells become resistant to its physiological pathways. Either way, the resulting effect is similar to that of Type 1 diabetes, wherein the underlying issue is a general inability to control blood glucose levels.

Also, Type 2 diabetes is a far more prevalent form of the disease; it is estimated to affect over 400 million people worldwide, or between 90 and 95% of the total diabetic population.

Additionally, far more risk factors are associated with Type 2 diabetes than there are with Type 1. Several of the most prominent of these factors include: weight (obesity); a high sugar diet combined with inactivity; family history/genetics; ethnicity (African-Americans, Hispanics, and American Indians are especially susceptible, though the reason is unknown); and age (people over 45 are far more likely to develop the disease).

Conventional Non CBD Treatment Methods

In both Type 1 and Type 2 diabetes, an inability for glucose to be absorbed into the body's cells results in it building up to dangerously high levels in the bloodstream. This results in the severe, potentially life-threatening symptoms that are most often associated with the disease. Some of these symptoms include:

Heart and blood vessel disease

Nerve damage

Stroke

Kidney disease

34

Vision problems

In short, there aren't many areas of the body that go unaffected by the physiological detriments of diabetes, and unless the disease is monitored closely on a daily basis, the average diabetic will have a lifespan between 10 and 15 years shorter than the average person's.

Fortunately, conventional medications have gotten to the point where diabetics – if they keep track of their glucose levels rigorously and maintain an appropriate diet – can lead a rather normal lifestyle.

Since they can't produce it on their own, most Type 1 diabetics will be prescribed insulin either in the form of shots that they have to self-administer, or in the form of a pump which automatically monitors blood glucose levels and injects the hormone as needed.

While these forms of treatment are state of the art, they're by no means 100% effective; even the most responsible of diabetics can find it difficult to avoid the dangerous conse☐uences of irregular glucose levels.

And not to mention, without top of the line health insurance, treatments like insulin pumps are far too expensive for the average individual to consider; most, in fact, are resorted to pricking blood from their finger to monitor sugar levels, and self-administering insulin shots through hypodermic needles.

In the case of Type 2 diabetes, individuals who are able to get by without having to take insulin shots will most likely be prescribed a pharmaceutical drug like Metformin or Avandia, which aid in the ability to properly regulate glucose.

However, as is far too common with these kinds of prescription meds, a range of severe side effects is often produced, as is a monthly medical bill that can seemingly be as cumbersome as the side effects themselves.

This is why thousands of diabetics in recent years have been more than willing to try alternative treatment options like CBD oil. Even if it can replace one of their prescription medications, it's generally more than worth it.

Not to mention, the general improvement in quality of life for diabetics that've added CBD to their treatment regimen has been consistent nearly across the board.

CBD OIL FOR DIABETES: WHAT THE RESEARCH HAS SHOWN

Like we mentioned earlier, in the world of medicine, anecdotal evidence can only go so far.

So regardless of the fact that many diabetics use CBD oil every day of their lives to help manage their condition, a lot of physicians will be wary to recommend it as a treatment unless they can point to the exact physiological reasons as to why it's beneficial.

Fortunately, along with its treatment potential for cancer and nervous disorders, CBD oil for diabetes has been one of the most thoroughly researched areas of medicinal cannabis.

Dr. Raphael Mechoulam, a research scientist out of the Hebrew University of Jerusalem, points to the fact that naturally-occurring CBD receptors occur throughout the human body – from the brain and nervous tissues, to organs and immune cells. And one of the organs where he's found the receptors to be highly prevalent?

THE PANCREAS.

In fact, endocannabinoid receptors (namely CB-1 receptors) have been found specifically in the organ's islet cells – the exact location where insulin is produced. And what's more, the stimulus of these receptors in the islet cells has already shown to have direct links to insulin production.

Now, regardless of how intriguing the research is, we simply cannot sit here and say that endocannabinoid receptors are directly responsible for the production of insulin, or that CBD is a cure for diabetes in any way shape or form. While it's possible that the receptors may play a crucial role in insulin's production, much more research will have to be done in order to pinpoint the physiological mechanisms and exact chemical pathways that are responsible for doing so.

We will say, though, that preliminary studies of CBD for diabetes have been so promising, it's led to American Journal of Medicine's Dr. Joseph Alpert to call on the DEA and the National Institute of Health (NIH) for increased funding and collaboration on it's continued research.

And moreover, the National Organization for the Reform of Marijuana Laws (NORML) has gone so far as to suggest that endocannabinoids may be "the most important physiologic system involved in establishing and maintaining human health," based on their central role in regulating homeostasis, which is the body's ability to maintain normative operating conditions in spite of harmful stimuli.

CBD FOR DIABETES: HOW IT CAN HELP TREAT UNDERLYING MEDICAL CONDITIONS

What's been even more concrete than research on CBD's role in insulin production, though, has been research on its ability to help treat and prevent common medical conditions associated with diabetes.

One of the most prominent factors associated with the development of insulin resistance in Type 2 diabetes is chronic inflammation related to obesity. The excessive presence of fatty tissue in obese Type 2 diabetics drastically limits the efficiency of glucose metabolism, which in turn results in high levels of sugar building up in the bloodstream. The specific anti-inflammatory properties of CBD, however, have long been known to directly combat glucose metabolic disorders and improve overall metabolism.

Nerve damage is another condition commonly associated with diabetes. In many instances diabetics will have very limited sensation in their lower extremities, and in severe cases, amputations of the leg(s) are often necessary. This is due to a lack of sufficient blood flow, which eventually results in the breakdown of tissue and the increased risk for infection. CBD, in turn, is a federally patented neuroprotectant, and has been shown to reduce infarcts (areas of dead tissue due to lack of blood flow) by up to 30%.

Likewise, there have been dozens of other publications as well that have showed great promise in the role of CBD as a treatment for diabetes, including studies on retinopathy (a disorder of the eyes) and diabetic cardiovascular dysfunction.

In short, the medical potential and therapeutic benefits of CBD oil for diabetes is nothing short of phenomenal; many thousands of diabetics use it every day to treat the disease and improve their overall quality of life, and many thousands more will continue to do so in the future in light of increased research and improved information.

And lastly, on a side note, it's important to point out that CBD oil will not get you high – unlike whole plant marijuana, it contains hardly any traces of THC, which is the specific cannabinoid responsible for the psychoactive properties of the drug.

CBD oils can range in terms of their overall concentrations of the active cannabinoid; not all tinctures are the same, and different dosages will be required depending on the specific oil that you end up using (although the proper dosage will always be labeled on the bottle).

Likewise, CBD oil is no guaranteed solution for all diabetics; while the majority of patients do find it highly therapeutic, it's certainly more effective for some than it is for others. As is always the case, it's important to do your own research, and if possible, speak with a professional about some possible tinctures that might be appropriate for you and your specific condition.

CHAPTER 6

CBD HEMP OIL CURES EPILEPSY

There has been a dramatic rise in news attention to medicinal cannabis in 2013, with reports on CNN, ABC, CBS, and local publications about high-cannabidiol cannabis oil effectively controlling the symptoms of rare epileptic conditions like Dravet syndrome, Doose syndrome, infantile spasms, cortical dysplasia, and more. These diseases can cause hundreds to thousands of seizures a week, while also impairing development in a number of other ways. For families with children suffering from such conditions, the challenges are overwhelming. Due to the extremely complex nature of Dravet and related syndromes, traditional pharmaceuticals are ineffective and often make the problems worse. With no other hope, families have turned to high-CBD cannabis oil, which is proving to work with miraculous efficacy.

To clarify, high-CBD cannabis oil is non-psychoactive and apparently even more beneficial than high-THC cannabis oil. Cannabidiol is another cannabinoid in the cannabis plant, like the more well-known psychoactive cannabinoid THC, with significant research suggesting neuroprotectant, anticancer, antidiabetic, anti-ischemic, antispasmodic, antipsychotic, and antibacterial properties, among others. Furthermore, cannabis oil is a type of extract from cannabis. Such oil contains large amounts of concentrated cannabinoids that can be orally ingested rather than smoked, preserving the medicinal compounds and allowing them to be delivered through digestive system, rather than the respiratory system.

The research suggests that CBD has panacea-like properties, and in practice, this is proving to be the case. On August 11th, 2013, Sanjay Gupta released a documentary on CNN about Charlotte Figi. Charlotte is a young Dravet syndrome patient who was having 300 grand mal seizures a week. No pharmaceuticals or dietary changes could do anything to reduce this number. Charlotte's parents learned about high-CBD cannabis oil, and after literally the first dose, Charlotte's seizures stopped. She now has less than three minor seizures a month. This case is nothing short of miraculous, and it's not isolated. Dr. Margaret Gedde, a Colorado Springs physician, is tracking 11 new patients of the Stanely brothers, the providers of Charlotte's high-CBD medicine. 9 of them have had 90-100% reductions in seizures, which again, is simply miraculous.

The epileptic conditions that CBD is proving to be effective against are extremely complex, and not even the most powerful, well researched pharmaceuticals have been capable of inducing any healing. Yet high-CBD cannabis oil is immediately and potently reducing symptoms, with the only side effects being systemically beneficial - more energy, better learning, improved behavior, and more.

It should not be surprising that results like these have been going on for years. Just like research shows cannabinoids are therapeutically effective against epilepsy, there is research suggesting they can eliminate cancers and control other serious diseases. And in practice, for epilepsy and these other conditions, the results are translating to humans. People have been reliably eliminating cancers for years and mitigating diseases like diabetes, Crohn's, fibromyalgia, heart disease, chronic pain, multiple sclerosis, and more. This is as serious as it gets, and more attention must be brought to this issue.

CHAPTER 7

CBD HEMP OIL HARDENS BONE

Another research paper has just been published that shows how cbd oil can help to contain the brittle bone disease, osteoporosis. Scientists at the Institute of Medical Sciences, University of Aberdeen, UK have discovered how a non-psychoactive compound in cannabis, cannabidiol oil helps to maintain bone strength.

The endocannabinoid system is a group of cell receptors that are activated by a group of endogenous lipids as well as compounds derived from the cannabis plant. The cannabinoid receptors are involved in a variety of physiological processes including appetite control, pain, memory and mood. Recent research has shown that the endocannabinoid system also has a strong influence on bone metabolism, as the receptors are well represented on osteoclasts - cells whose principal function is to resorb (thin out) bone.

Bone is an active, living tissue that is being continuously formed, remodeled and shaped in response to both physical and physiological needs of the body. Bone matrix consists primarily of the macronutrients calcium, magnesium and phosphate and is the material that makes up both the dense parts of the bone and the bone marrow framework. Many people still believe that if one eats foods rich in these minerals then they will avoid developing osteoporosis. Epidemiological and other evidence suggests that this is not necessarily the case.

When it comes to bone health and disease the integrated processes that control the formation and resorption bone are just as important as the availability of calcium, magnesium and phosphate.

The formation and resorbtion of bone matrix is controlled by two main cell types:

1) Osteoblasts are bone cells that are responsible for the formation of bone matrix

2) Osteoclasts are modified white blood cells responsible for the resorption of bone tissue.

These two cell types are controlled by a complex set of signaling hormones, proteins and cell receptors that respond to the ever-changing demands on bone tissue and other physiological processes. If there are too many osteoclasts, or if these cells become overactive, they will resorb more matrix than the osteoblasts can produce. A

49

predominance of osteoclast activity results in the bone becoming less dense - the principal characteristic of the clinical condition known as osteoporosis.

The Aberdeen researchers have discovered that cannabidiol binds to a specific cannabinoid receptor on the bone-resorbing osteoblast cells. By so doing it inhibits these cells from resorbing the bone matrix - thereby helping to prevent further weakening of the bones.

This is not the first time that plant compounds have been shown to influence bone metabolism in favour of stronger bones. In January 2009 researchers at Oklahoma State University in the USA found that, even in the presence of oxidative stress and systemic inflammation, polyphenols derived from plums inhibit the action of the bone-softening osteoclasts but enhance the generation and activity of bone-building osteoblasts.

CHAPTER 8

CBD HEMP OIL CURES BACK PAIN

Chronic back pain can only really be fully understood by people that suffer from chronic back pain. Those who don't suffer from chronic back pain can merely sympathize. There are various treatments available for chronic back pain, all of which will only help up to a certain point. In the following chapter we are going to discuss CBD for back pain.

And be aware that most medications for severe pain can cause damage to internal organs. The most severe cases of chronic back pain nearly always end up being treated by means of surgery after neuropathy and physiotherapy fail.

Common cause of Back Pain

Intervertebral discsIntervertebral discs are the cartilage discs located between the vertebrae in the spinal cord of mammals.

It is their purpose to absorb shock before it reaches the vertebrae, and to improve mobility of the spine.

But when these intervertebral discs become degenerated they can cause havoc for the sufferer.

The degeneration of these discs is believed to be the number one cause of chronic back pain and neck pain.

And while around 25% of the population goes burdened by uncontested signs of IVD degeneration, there still is no sign of an effective treatment and/or therapy.

Contributing factors such as oxygen deficiency, a lack of essential sugars and water, aging and inflammation of the painful region are considered to be the main causes of degeneration of the intervertebral discs.

It was reported by the Institute of Medicine of The National Academies that 100 million Americans have to live with chronic pain.

And more specifically with chronic back pain. Medical researchers have been working endlessly to find a safer and more cost effective treatment than NSAIDS.

Using CBD Oil

In reply to the □uestion whether CBD oil will help managing pain, the answer would be that according to research there is a high degree of probability that this would be the case.

As far as symptoms go, acute or chronic pain is the most common denominator. No matter what the ailment, pain is most likely involved.

53

Various disorders, including Diabetic Neuropathy, Fibromyalgia and others, cause pain that simply will not subside. Whether from the primary or central nervous system, the pain is not easily controlled by regular pain meds.

However, certain studies involving the treatment of pain with CBD (Cannabidiol) oil intake on pain management do exist.

CHAPTER 9

CBD HEMP OIL CURES ARTHRITIS

What is Arthritis?

Rheumatoid arthritis is a chronic progressive disease that causes inflammation in joints. As a result, it causes immobility and painful deformity in feet, wrists, fingers, and ankles.

In this disease, there is inflammation like swelling, pain and heat that affects joints and also body organs. Most commonly affected areas are hands, knees, and feet. It usually affects between the age of 25 and 45 but it can also affect children even toddlers.

CBD for Arthritis: Causes and symptoms

When rheumatoid arthritis affects a person, it attacks normal tissue components as invading pathogens cause inflammation.

The inflammation attacks the lining of the joints and then spreads to cartilage and bone while causing destruction therein and making joints immobile and deformed.

There are environmental and genetic factors involved in this reaction.

Symptoms vary from one person to another and it may include swelling, pain in joints, persistent fatigue, stiff joints especially in the morning, sleep difficulties owing to pain and weakness in muscles.

Making a diagnose is not so hard as the disease shows itself over a few months. Only an expert can tell after complete examination and check-up. Blood tests also help identify rheumatoid arthritis factor that is present in almost 80 percent of people suffering from rheumatoid.

There are certain factors that increase the chances of developing rheumatoid arthritis. These are ages (25 to 45), gender (three-□uarter patients are female), family history of rheumatoid arthritis, ethnicity (Americans, Caucasians have a higher risk) and obesity.

There are ways through proper methods and techni□ues to alleviate the discomfort.. Physiotherapy that involves heat, cold and exercises to relieve stiffness and pain is an effective way.

Rest and occupational therapy are also effective. Drugs are also available that include NSAIDs (non-steroidal anti-inflammatory drugs) to treat inflammation but these have side effects.

Corticosteroids are also used that suppress immune reaction. DMARDs (disease modifying anti-rheumatic drugs) slow down the progress of the disease but they can bring about serious side effects.

CBD for Arthritis: CBD Oil as a Treatment?

CBD-A-Cannabinoil CBD oil has shown lots of improvement in the treatment of arthritis. According to research, cannabidiol helps reduce pain and inflammation caused by arthritis of all types like Rheumatoid arthritis, gout, osteoarthritis and other types of inflammatory joint conditions.

Cannabidiol (CBD) is a compound that is found in cannabis and is also called hemp oil. CBD is also taken from medical marijuana plants.

Doctors have successfully treated rheumatoid arthritis with CBD oil that gives relief from inflammation and pain. According to a study conducted in 2006 where patients used CBD oil for a five-week period.

They experienced improvement in less pain and inflammation. It also slowed down the progression of rheumatoid arthritis considerably. Patients who are fed up with drugs and want to go for a natural treatment of this disease can use CBD oil according to the instructions given by experts.

CHAPTER 10

CBD HEMP OIL CURES FIBROMYALGIA

What is fibromyalgia?

Fibromyalgia is a chronic disease characterized by symptoms of chronic pain, insomnia, migraines, fatigue, joint pain, and irritable bowel issues.

People with fibromyalgia suffer from an increased sensitivty to pain. This is thought to be caused by an abnormal functioning of pain signals in the central nervous system.

Commonly used treatments for fibromyalgia are pain relievers like NSAIDs and opioids, muscle relaxants, and sleep aids.

Some patients are instead opting for CBD and THC products to treat their fibromylagia. They are finding that cannabis products are safer and have less side effects than the prescription medications they were previously using.

Why does CBD work for fibromyalgia?

While more data is needed to confirm this theory, it is thought that fibromyalgia is one of the conditions caused by an endocannabinoid deficiency or dysregulation.

An endocannabinoid deficiency/dysregulation is when a person has a poorly functioning endocannabinoid system. This results from having abnormal levels of endocannabinoids.

If a person's body doesn't produce a sufficient amount of endocannabinoids, they will be more sensitive to pain. Endocannabinoids are neuro-modulators and they regulate our perception of pain. Without a sufficient supply of endocannabinoids, the endocannabinoid system cannot properly do its job of maintaining balance in the body – and thus people with fibromyalgia experience more pain than what is usual.

CBD can help our endocannabinoid system. CBD interferes with the body's natural process of breaking down endocannabinoids. This is a good thing – supplementing with CBD can increase our levels of endocannabinoids and take care of the deficiency a person may have.

What are the effects of using CBD for fibromyalgia?

People using cannabis medicine for fibromyalgia are reporting the following benefits:

Improved mood

Pain relief

Improved sleep

Less inflammation

Reduction or cessation of prescription medication and henceforth a decrease in negative side effects.

What are the side effects of using CBD for fibromyalgia?

Generally CBD has few negative side effects. However it can be sedating for some people, especially if it is used in high doses. Always start with a low dose if you are new to CBD and work your way up. It's a good idea to take CBD the first few times in the comfort of your home, when you do not have to drive, in case you do experience some negative side effects.

How should I use CBD for fibromyalgia?

People with fibromyalgia symptoms are finding the best delivery methods to be vaporizing or sublingual tinctures because of the speed of the effects from these methods.

CBD dominant products, THC dominant products, and a combination of CBD/THC products are all useful for helping with fibromyalgia. When used in combination, THC and CBD have been found to be particularly effective for pain relief.

If you are completely new to using cannabis, it's always best to start with a CBD dominant product as it will be non-psychoactive and less likely to cause negative side effects.

5 – 10 mg of CBD is a good, low dose to start with. Increase the dose as needed until you reach the desired effect.

What terpenes are good for helping with fibromyalgia?

The properties of certain terpenes are useful for helping with fibromyalgia symptoms. These terpenes work synergistically with CBD. Try to find products with lab results that show higher amounts of these terpenes:

B-caryophyllene – anti-inflammatory and pain relieving

Pinene – anti-inflammatory

Linalool – Pain relieving and relaxing

CHAPTER 11

CBD HEMP OIL CURES SCLEROSIS

Do you happen to be a victim of Multiple Sclerosis? Are you looking

for treatment options for yourself? Then you have landed on the right page. Assuming that you are a victim of the unfortunate medical condition, it is highly unlikely that you haven't heard of cannabis as a treatment option. In this report we will discuss CBD and Multiple Sclerosis.

The use of CBD oil for the purpose of treating multiple sclerosis has been spreading at a tremendous pace. We have taken the liberty of mentioning how does CBD work to treat multiple sclerosis in the first place. Without further ado, let's take a closer look at its mode of action.

CBD and Multiple Sclerosis: Some Tips

Tips: Last but not the least, we would like to mention some tips or rather a schedule of consuming CBD for the treatment of your multiple sclerosis:

Make sure that you are taking a pill of CBD during the day in order to keep the symptoms of your medical condition under control without putting yourself at the risk of getting high either

Vaporize high CBD cannabis and it'll enable you to relieve the pain and associated symptoms. It would be a wise decision however, to not drive right after the consumption

Consume a CBD rich edible before you go to sleep to keep the inflammation and pain at bay during sleep. Consumption during the day will disable you from driving or working properly.

If you happen to be one lucky individual who is located in an area that sells cannabis juice commonly, it'll be a commendable idea to consume it as much as you can afford.

CHAPTER 12

IS CBD HEMP OIL LEGAL?

In a context of research and legality in many countries, the percentage of cannabidiol usage by inhalation, oral drops, topicals, concentrates and food supplements is increasing day by day. On the other hand, there are those who are already working to define cannabidiol under the term drug, which could completely stop the current free trade? In this chapter we are going to explain whether CBD oil is legal or not.

New revelations about CBD Oil's therapeutic capabilities have made cannabidiol more popular.

Nowadays, many entrepreneurs and consumers join in what appears to be a real revolution in the use of cannabis components that do not cause a high. In not too distant future, CBD will become an essential source for the composition of health food products, in food supplements and also in the composition of pharmaceutical drugs.

A Drug Or A Food Supplement – Regulated or Freely available

If it's finally decided that the CBD should not be listed on global drug laws or otherwise defined as a medicinal substance, a real revolution in the field is expected. If approved as a dietary supplement, cannabidiol will become a component consumed daily by millions of people around the globe. Such a change also has broad industrial implications for opening new factories and creating jobs.

On the other hand, if it's decided that the CBD is completely medical, its use will be strictly prohibited by anyone who is not a recognized pharmaceutical company with a specific license to use, market and sell the substance after having been proven in clinical trials and regulatory files.

CBD declared as Supplement not as medicine

Pending a new announcment, cbd continues to be considered a dietry supplement as long as the companies that sell it do not declare it as a medical product. This allows the trade of cbd products to continue and the grow and spread around the globe, particulary in Europe.

Over the past 2-3 years, cbd has taken off. And in parallel with the developement of thechnologies to separate the molecule from the plant in laboratory, medical cannabis companies around the world have started marketing cannabis varieties.

The reactions were constructive, and very swiftly the flower became like green oil, which is now consumed daily by millions of people around the world, as part of a daily diet.

IS CBD Oil legal?

Yes, in most countries of the world CBD Hemp Oil is legal. This is a good news and we can use the CBD benefits for ourselves. It's because of the simple reason, that what makes cannabis illegal is THC and not CBD.

In the international legislative text about how to deal with cannabis is written, that for the people in the States which have associated to this international prohibition against cannabis, are the following products of cannabis illegal to buy and sell:

The definition of this convention is provided above, serves to explain the concept of cannabis:

Cannabis refers to the flower or inflorescence tips of the hemp plant. The hemp seeds and hemp leaves are so far that the flowers were separated from it.

The resin of the cannabis plant in extracted form, whatever you want to call it.

Cannabis plant refers to any genus or species of the hemp plant.

Excluded are plants, wherein the THC limit of 0,2 % is not exceeded.

In Fact, CBD Oil which contains CBD as main ingredient is extracted from Hemp Plants with a concentration of THC lower than 0,2 %.

71

The following list is a list of countries that we know does allow CBD Oil from Hemp:

United States

Argentina

Austria

Belgium

Belize

Brazil

Bulgaria

Canada

Chile

China

Colombia

Costa Rica

Croatia

Cyprus

Czech Republic

Denmark

England

Estonia

Finland

France

Georgia

Germany

Greece

Guam

Guatemala

Hong Kong

Hungary

Iceland

India

Ireland

Italy

Latvia

Lithuania

Luxembourg

Malta

Netherlands

Netherlands Antilles

Northern Ireland

Norway

Paraguay

Peru

Poland

Portugal

Puerto Rico

Romania

Russia

Scotland

Slovak Republic

Slovenia

South Africa

Sweden

Switzerland

U.S. Virgin Islands

United Kingdom

Uruguay

Wales.

If you do not live in one of these countries, CBD Oil extracted from a Cannabis Sativa Variety with a THC content less then 0,2% (Hemp) may be not legal. But you should inform yourself about the law in your country before ordering.

Another step in public recognition

The entry of Cannabidiol into the world of legal trade has taken an important step this year (October 2017) with the World Agency against Doping in Sport (WADA AMA) which announced the list of 2018 in which CBD will be withdrawn from the list of drugs that are banned in the sport.

The non-hepatic cannabis component, which has excellent anti-inflammatory and pain-relieving effects, can now be an integral part of the athletes' training menu.

CBD is worth much more than just the money

CBD sales are expected to reach $ 500 million by the end of 2017, 200 million more compared to 2015. The Hemp Business Journal estimates that by 2021 the United States CBD market is going to reach $ 2.1 billion, As reported some time ago on the popular website Forbes

The costs of pure raw CBD in kilograms, of course vary, depending on the □uality of the final product. Some laboratories produce cannabidiol with a purity level less than 90% and others reach the 99% level. The price or maybe cost gap between these 2 products is enormous.

In addition to the huge sums of money and the huge value of the molecule, its lack of psychoactive activity and its health benefits in each mode of consumption creates a new industry around cannabidiol and will allow the creation of new factories, stores and thousands of jobs. This could happen soon.

Despite fears of redefining cannabidiol as a drug that would transfer its rights to pharmaceutical companies, the industry assumes that we can no longer backtrack.

CHAPTER 13

WHAT ARE THE VARIOUS TYPES OF HEMP OIL

Hemp oils can be broken down into 3 different types:

Hemp Seed Oil (Unrefined and Refined)

CBD Hemp Oil

Hemp Essential Oil

All these oils are both extracted from the plant and processed in different ways. More importantly, all these oils offer different benefits. Understanding what properties each of these oils have will help you understand which hemp oil to shop for the next time you're looking to try one.

HEMP SEED OIL (UNREFINED AND REFINED)

Hemp seed oil comes from the seeds of the hemp plant. There are two different ways hemp seed oil can be processed:

UNREFINED, COLD-PRESSED HEMP SEED OIL

This oil is green in color with a nutty flavor. Cold pressed hemp oil preserves hemp's nutritious content, so it is often called "Nature's most perfectly balanced oil".

Unrefined, cold-pressed hemp oil is processed in minimal heat. This means that the oil has not been bleached or deodorized. A lot of unrefined oils are also called "virgin", "extra virgin", "raw", or "pure". This also means that unrefined oil has a much shorter shelf life and should be stored in the refrigerator once opened. The oil can also start smelling odd when it gets closer to its expiration date. When you hear someone complaining about the foul odor from a hemp seed oil they just bought, you can assume that the bottle was in storage for a while. In this case, we'd recommend you reach out to the manufacturer to ask for a refund and/or exchange.

REFINED HEMP SEED OIL

Refined oil is clear and colorless. It doesn't have much flavor and also lacks the natural vitamins and antioxidants that hemp is known for. That's because this oil is typically used as ingredients for body care products, fuel, lubricants, and even plastics.

This oil has been bleached and deodorized. That is why refined oil has a much longer shelf life, and can be used in body care products. As Dr. Bronners, the biggest hemp soap maker, advocates hemp oil for its superfatting ingredients. They have been using hemp oil in their soaps for over 150 years for its amazing Essential Fatty Acid (EFA) content, which essentially means that the soap is smoother and a great moisturizer.

CBD HEMP OIL

CBD (Cannabidiol) is a a non psychoactive cannabinoid derived from hemp plants mainly for medical use. CBD oils are known to provide safe and effective relief even for patients who suffer from seizures, epilepsy, or cancer. Even though CBD shows much promise, it is still a largely grey market that is still heavily regulated. With the recent legalization in certain states, it is one of the fastest growing applications in the hemp industry.

Since cultivation in the US is still in its infancy, most CBD oil is imported into the US and then examined for purity and quality before being sold commercially. The regulation behind the CBD oil products are still largely grey and customers should be very cautious of buying CBD products without proper guidance.

HEMP ESSENTIAL OIL

Hemp essential oil comes from the upper leaves and flowers of the hemp plant. The leaves and flowers are then steam distilled to capture the pure essence of the plant. Pale yellow to light green in color with a a highly concentrated therapeutic aroma. It takes over fifty pounds to make 1 ounce of hemp essential oil. It is also one of the most expensive oils in the world – and contains no THC or CBD.

Hemp essential oil is well known for its essential oil aroma and therapeutic abilities on the central nervous system. It helps to release stress and relax the body. Its earthy, peppery and faintly sweet scent is alluring and sensual; blending perfectly with other fragrances to perfect the art of aromatherapy.

There aren't many brands in the US that offer hemp essential oil, but there are a few uni□ue brands that are using hemp essential oil in candles and massage oil to promote its therapeutic properties.

WHY IT MATTERS

As hemp oil becomes increasingly popular among active people looking for a healthy supplement or patients considering a medical alternative, it's important that we know which oil offers what benefits. Taking hemp seed oil with the hopes that it'll help you "relax" or get rid of chronic pain can only be discouraging. At best, you'll experience a few placebo effects.

So if you're looking to try hemp oil, make sure to learn what type of hemp oil will best fit your needs. Proactively share your knowledge with your friends and family so they aren't confused about the benefits that hemp oil offers.

CHAPTER 14

THINGS TO CONSIDER WHEN BUYING HEMP SEED OIL

1. What does "Cold Pressed" mean?

Typically, when you press seeds for oil, the temperature rises from the heat that's produced from the friction caused by pressing and grinding. When the heat rises too high, this makes the oil lose a lot of its value. By cold pressing, presses are re☐uired to maintain a much lower temperature (less than 120 degrees Fahrenheit), which ensures that the oil retains the flavor, aroma, and nutritional value of the seed. That is why unrefined cold-pressed hemp maintains a green color, smells nutty, and contains all sorts of nutrition.

2. Refined vs Unrefined

Unrefined has a similar meaning to "cold-pressed" in that the oil is processed in minimal heat. But it also means that the oil has not been bleached or deodorized. A lot of unrefined oils are also called "virgin", "extra virgin", "raw", or "pure". This also means that unrefined oil has a much shorter shelf life and the oil can start smelling odd when it gets closer to its expiration date. Refined oil, on the other hand, has been bleached and/or deodorized. That is why refined oil has a much longer shelf life. If you're ever in doubt, try observing and smelling the oil. If the oil is clear, doesn't taste like anything, and doesn't have any scent, it is most likely refined.

3. How are you using it?

Before buying hemp oil, it's important to decide why you're buying it. How do you plan on using the hemp oil? Will you use it as a dressing or additive to your daily diet? Do you plan on using it for your skin? Depending on what your answer is, you can tailor what type of hemp oil to buy. If you are looking to eat (or drink) hemp oil for its nutritional benefits, we recommend checking out the price & reviews section to see what unrefined hemp oil is the best fit for you. If you are considering hemp oil for your skin, there are many other options you could consider. Unrefined hemp oil is used to make some amazing body care products.

4. Capsules or Li☐uid oil?

Hemp oil is typically sold in bottles that you can store in the fridge. But if you are simply looking to "eat" hemp oil for its nutritional benefits, some brands offer hemp oil in capsules. Capsules is advantageous in that they have a longer shelf life and they don't have to be refrigerated, unlike regular hemp oil. You can simply take them daily like you would your vitamin pills. But if you would rather enjoy your daily hemp oil with your shakes or salad, getting a regular hemp oil bottle offers you more variety in ways to eating it.

5. Read reviews

The hemp seed oil market is becoming saturated with a lot of new brands looking to take advantage of this growing health product. If this is your first time shopping for hemp products, it might be difficult to compare the different products and decide which one offers the best value and quality.

CHAPTER 15

HOW DO YOU MAKE CBD HEMP OIL

There are a number of ways of extracting CBD from any of these varieties of cannabis. If the plant you start with contains only CBD (like industrial hemp or a high-CBD cannabis strain); there are multiple extraction methods which are very simple and require little equipment.

The most common methods use some type of solvent. This can be a liquid solvent, CO2, or an oil solvent. If the plant material you start with contains THC as well as CBD (such as smokable cannabis), the process to separate CBD from other cannabinoids is more complex and generally requires professional equipment. To avoid getting too technical, let's look mainly at extraction methods for CBD-only plants.

Li□uid Solvents

In this method, plant material like flowers and trim are put into a container. Li□uid solvent (usually butane, isopropyl alcohol, hexane, or ethanol) is run through the plant matter to strip it of cannabinoids and flavours and transfer them into the li□uid. Then, the li□uid is evaporated away from this mixture to leave only concentrated chemicals and flavours in the form of an oil.

Benefits of this method are many, it is the most simple, e□uipment-free, and inexpensive way to extract CBD, but not without some downsides. One concern is that solvents can leave traces of impurities in the finished CBD oil (meticulous processing methods and the right solvent can minimise this).

Also, some li□uid solvents remove chlorophyll from the plant along with cannabinoids and flavours, giving the finished oil a greener colour and more bitter taste.

However, because these negative effects can usually be countered by adjusting specifics in the process, this remains the most common method for CBD extraction.

C02 Extraction

Carbon Dioxide (C02) is a unique molecule that can function as any state of matter— solid, liquid, or gas— depending on the pressure and temperature it is kept under. Because variables like pressure and temperature have to be kept very specific in a C02 extraction, this extraction method is usually done with a piece of equipment called a 'closed-loop extractor'.

This machine has three chambers: the first chamber holds solid, pressurised C02 (commonly known as 'dry ice'), the second chamber contains dry plant material and the third chamber separates the finished product.

When performing the extraction, the solid CO_2 from the first chamber is pumped into the second with the plant material. This second chamber is kept at a specific pressure and temperature which causes the CO_2 to behave more like a liquid (although it's actually somewhere between a liquid and gas in this state, referred to as supercritical CO_2) so that it runs through the plant material and extracts chemicals and flavours, much like in the liquid solvent process. Then, the CO_2-cannabinoid mixture is pumped into a third chamber where it is kept at an even lower pressure and higher temperature so that the CO_2 gas rises to the top of the chamber while the oils containing chemicals and flavours from the plant material fall to the bottom to be collected for consumption.

There are many benefits of this method. It doesn't require a long evaporation process like a liquid solvent extraction and there is minimal risk of contaminants in the finished product.

Because this method carefully controls temperature and pressure, it can also be used to separate CBD from cannabis also containing THC.

CBD extracts from the plant at a lower temperature and pressure than THC, so careful adjustment of the pressure and temperature in the second chamber can isolate the specific cannabinoid you want to extract. Closed-loop extractor systems are very pricey, however, which is why this type of extraction is generally only used by professional CBD producers.

Oil Extraction

Using oils, especially olive oil, to extract cannabinoids from hemp and cannabis is a practice that dates back to biblical times or even earlier.

Many home-producers who make their own CBD products still employ this simple extraction method. First, raw plant material must be decarboxylated, or heated to a specific temperature for a certain length of time to activate the chemicals in the plant. Plant material is then added to olive oil and heated to 100°C for 1-2 hours to extract the cannabinoids. With this method, the olive oil cannot be evaporated away after the process, so users must consume much higher quantities of this type of extracted oil than the highly-concentrated oil produced by other methods. Infused olive oil is also highly perishable, and so must be stored in cold, dark place.

While these are currently the most common methods in which CBD is extracted from cannabis or hemp; technology in this exciting new field is constantly updating, so new methods will surely be seen in the coming years as the industry expands.

Each extraction method is best suited to specific circumstances: whether you are a company or an individual, for what type of product you are extracting CBD, desired flavour, strength and consistency all play a part in which method should be chosen.

CHAPTER 16

HOW YOU CAN USE HEMP OIL FOR HEALTH AND BEAUTY?

Alleviate dry skin. Rub the oil directly onto dry, cracked skin. For a deep conditioning treatment for hands and feet, massage in the oil, then wear socks or gloves overnight to let it work its magic.

Strengthen nails and heal cuticles. Massage a small amount of hemp oil directly into nails and cuticles, great for both fingernails and toenails.

Remove makeup. Oil follows the "like dissolves like" rule, which means that hemp oil will dissolve the oils and waxes in makeup, especially in stubborn eye makeup. Gently rub a small amount of oil into the makeup and wipe with a cotton ball or a soft tissue.

Mask overnight. Massage hemp oil into cleansed facial skin before bedtime.

Steam facial skin. Massage a tablespoon of oil into the skin on your dry, clean face, massaging for several minutes. Then lay a hot (not scalding) damp washcloth over your face and let it sit until it cools. Wipe with the washcloth. Repeat with another hot washcloth until all the oil is wiped off. Washing your face afterwards is optional.

Condition hair. Before shampooing, massage a tablespoon or so of hemp oil into your scalp and let it sit for about 10 minutes. Afterwards, shampoo as normal. You might find you don't need conditioner.

Reduce acne. This may sound crazy, but this oil actually reduces acne. Massage hemp oil into problem areas and work it in gently for several minutes. The oil will actually draw out sebum plugs that cause whiteheads, blackheads, and even cysts. Do this daily during breakouts.

Relieve eczema. A 2005 study found that 2 tablespoons of dietary hemp seed oil consumed daily may help relieve the effects of atopic dermatitis, or eczema.

Support overall health. Eat it. You can eat it straight and enjoy its nutty flavor or you can put it in salad dressings, as a butter replacement on toast, rice, potatoes, vegetables...it's delicious! Keep in mind that pure hemp seed oil cannot be used for high-heat cooking. It has a low smoke point and will totally break down even at a moderate heat, at which point all nutritional benefits are lost

SUMMARY

"Take Control of Your Health Naturally"

What is CBD Hemp Oil?

CBD, also called Cannabidiol, is just one of 85 different chemical compounds in marijuana plants. CBD Hemp Oil is derived from hemp, or cannabis grown with very little THC (often less than

0.3%). For the sake of this article we will refer to marijuana as cannabis grown for its psychoactive effects, and hemp as cannabis grown for its practical uses as a fiber. Marijuana is marketed for its THC content and hemp is utilized for its CBD content.

THC is the psychoactive or intoxicating compound found in cannabis plants whereas, CBD oil is not psychoactive or intoxicating and has shown strong signs of being an effective treatment for a variety of diseases and mental health disorders.

Where Can I Get CBD Hemp Oil?

Hemp oil is legal in all 50 states but the production of CBD Hemp Oil is not. Even though both come from marijuana, hemp oil is derived from sterile cannabis seeds, which are legal under the Controlled Substances Act. CBD Oil is derived from the plant's flowers which are not legal in some states. However, this doesn't stop the import of CBD oil made from industrialized hemp grown legally, which is why you're able to buy it legally on the internet.

You can find products containing hemp oil in the beauty section of your local retail store, but to get CBD Oil you'll either need to be in a state where it's legal to produce or purchase an import.

CBD Hemp Oil Health Benefits

CBD Oil has been shown to have surprisingly positive effects on a variety of diseases. Some of the Cannabidiol health benefits are:

Nausea treatment

Lowered anxiety

Pain relief

Improved mood

Lessening withdrawal symptoms

Seizure reduction

Stimulating appetite

CBD works by activating the body's serotonin (anti-depressant effect), vanilloid (pain relief), and adenosine (anti-inflammatory effect) receptors. How quickly you start to feel the results from CBD Oil depends on how it was ingested and your weight. Someone small who ingested the oil in spray form will feel the effects much faster than a larger person ingesting CBD in capsule form.

Different Forms of CBD Hemp Oil

CBD Hemp Oil can take on many different forms, including liquids, ointments, and sprays, and capsules. Most oils and sprays are used by putting the substance under your tongue. Ointments are used on and absorbed by the skin, and thirdly capsules are ingested. Those who don't like the taste of sprays or oils can defer to capsules. Capsules are a very convenient way to consume Cannabidiol, however you don't absorb as much CBD from a capsule as you do from an oil or spray put under your tongue.

CBD vape oil is the same as regular CBD Hemp Oil - it's just taken into the body in a different way. You just fill your vape pen with Cannabidiol and presto, you've got yourself a vape with health benefits.

CBD Oil sold online are not as potent as those medically prescribed for serious diseases but they can help with mood disorders, lower anxiety, and lessen pain caused by inflammation.

CBD Hemp Oil Side Effects

While not much research has been done yet on the side effects of CBD Oil, whether absorbed, swallowed as a capsule or inhaled through a CBD vape pen, the most commonly side effects reported are digestive issues, such as upset stomach and diarrhea, which are not very common.

Will CBD Hemp oil Show On a Drug Test?

Drug tests are looking for THC, not CBD, and because CBD doesn't produce any kind of high, employers really have no reason to look for it in the first place. So CBD Oil does not show up on a drug test. However, for this reason, make sure you purchase pure CBD oil with 0% THC.

Unique Benefits of Using Pure CBD Oil

No prescription re□uired: Even though they are more potent than regular CBD Oils, most pure CBD Oils do not re□uire a prescription.

0% THC: If you're worried about using a cannabis extract because you don't want to experience marijuana's psychoactive effects or fail a drug test, opt for pure CBD Oil. Containing no THC at all, it's the safest choice.

Fewer side effects: Pure CBD Oils are less likely to cause nausea and fatigue.

Purchase Cautions: How do you know if you are getting □uality CBD Hemp Oil?

Your first clue is usually price. If the price seems too cheap to be true, it probably is.

Always purchase from a reputable source. A company that is reputable will back their product and will not risk selling misrepresented items.

Another thing to look for is the way that the product is marketed. If you see CBD Hemp Oil online that claims to cure every ailment under the sun, it's also probably too good to be true.

The top products are made from organically grown hemp and have a CBD concentration over 20mg.

While the medicinal effects of Cannabidiol are great, keep your expectations of online brands realistic.

HOW MUCH CBD OIL SHOULD I TAKE?

To increase appetite in cancer patients: 2.5 milligrams of THC by mouth with or without 1 mg of CBD for six weeks

To treat chronic pain: 2.5-20 mg CBD by mouth for an average of 25 days.

To treat epilepsy: 200-300 mg of CBD by mouth daily.

To treat movement problems associated with Huntington's disease: 10 mg per kilogram of CBD by mouth daily for six weeks.

To treat sleep disorders: 40-160 mg CBD by mouth.

To treat multiple sclerosis symptoms: Cannabis plant extracts containing 2.5-120 milligrams of a THC-CBD combination by mouth daily for 2-15 weeks. A mouth spray might contain 2.7 milligrams of THC and 2.5 milligrams of CBD at doses of 2.5-120 milligram for up to eight weeks. Patients typically use eight sprays within any three hours, with a maximum of 48 sprays in any 24-hour period.

To treat schizophrenia: 40-1,280 mg CBD by mouth daily.

To treat glaucoma: a single CBD dose of 20-40 mg under the tongue. Doses greater than 40 mg may actually increase eye pressure.

To treat diabetis: CBD dosages can range anywhere from 10 mg to 200 mg per day.

If you are new to using CBD, always start low and go slow. A general starting dose of CBD is 10 mg, one to two times per day.

Talk to your doctor about adding CBD to your supplement routine. You can increase the dosage as much as you feel comfortable.

www.ingramcontent.com/pod-product-compliance
Lightning Source LLC
Chambersburg PA
CBHW051323220526
45468CB00004B/1475